The Pregnasaurus

Written by Jodi Neelin
Illustrated by Russell Neelin

Russell,
Thank you for seeing what was in my mind's eye
and bringing it to life in these illustrations.
And thank you for making me the most ungainly
yet deliriously happy Pregnasaurus!
I love you.

For my sweet Jenna,
Whom I adore with my whole heart.
I would do this a thousand times for you.

Some women are graceful in their pregnancies.
They glow and exude serenity with the promise
of the miraculous new life that grows inside them.
They are flawless, the essence of beauty,
and have never been more radiant.

Others... are not.

To every gigantic, clumsy, waddling,
acne-ridden, emotional, furry-faced, aching
barge with arms and legs, this one's for you!!

There was once a young woman,
Who did her own thing,
Like spend time with her friends, and go to karaoke bars and sing.

She and her husband
Would go out on dates;
It was common to find her at work until late.

But slowly she noticed
That things weren't quite right,
She was going to the bathroom at least three times a night.

She would sometimes get dizzy,
Her breasts felt like rock,
She had trouble staying up past eight o'clock.

Then one morning it hit her,
She just had an inkling,
Of the cause of the tiredness and two a.m. tinkling.

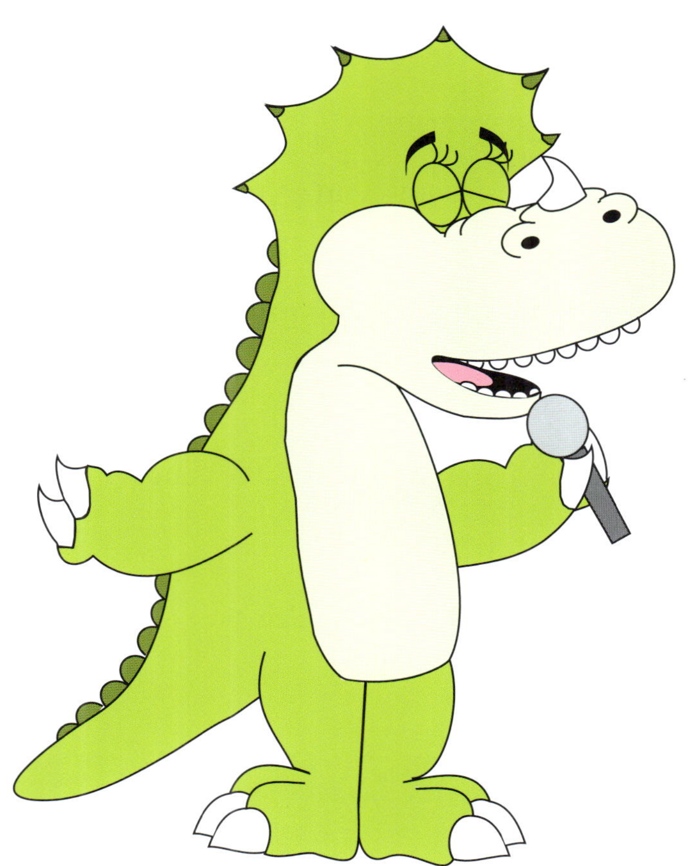

So she picked up a home kit
And peed on the stick,
And the second pink line showed up quick as a lick.

She knew in that instant
Her whole life would change
And it dawned on the woman why all was so strange.

And she gaped
At the pregnancy test she had bought.
"I'm going to be somebody's mother!!!" she thought.

So she went out
And purchased the tiniest socks,
And wrapped them inside of the tiniest box.

When her husband got home
She presented the box,
And then waited for him to interpret the socks.

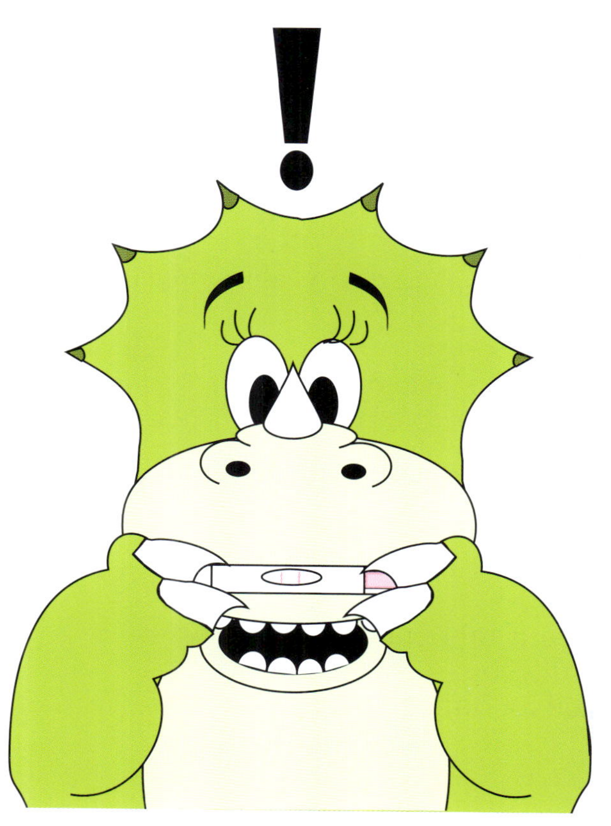

His face was confusion
As he tried to sift
Through the meaning of what was contained in this gift.

Then all of a sudden
He figured it out,
He felt so elated he wanted to shout.

But he was so overwhelmed
By the news she let out
That a stunned "Are you sure?" was the best he could spout.

When she showed him the test
The tears filmed on his eyes
He was quite overcome by this awesome surprise.

And so the young woman
Began to transform
As the world's newest Pregnasaurus was born.

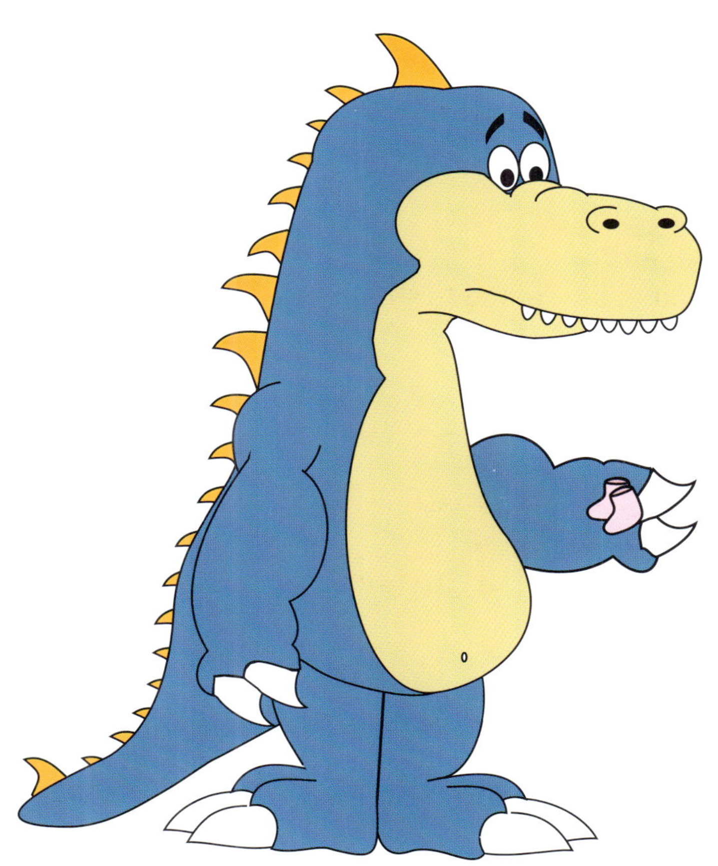

They bought all the books
About what to expect
And the baby equipment they'd have to collect.

Besides the odd symptoms
That had come about,
Being pregnant was not much to write home about.

But then the nausea hit
In the next few weeks,
"Peeeuw!" retched the Pregnasaurus, "Everything reeks!!"

She couldn't get past
Her intense sense of smell,
And thus spent the next while in olfactory hell.

The suggestion of food
Just about did her in,
And the look of it quivered her sensitive chin.

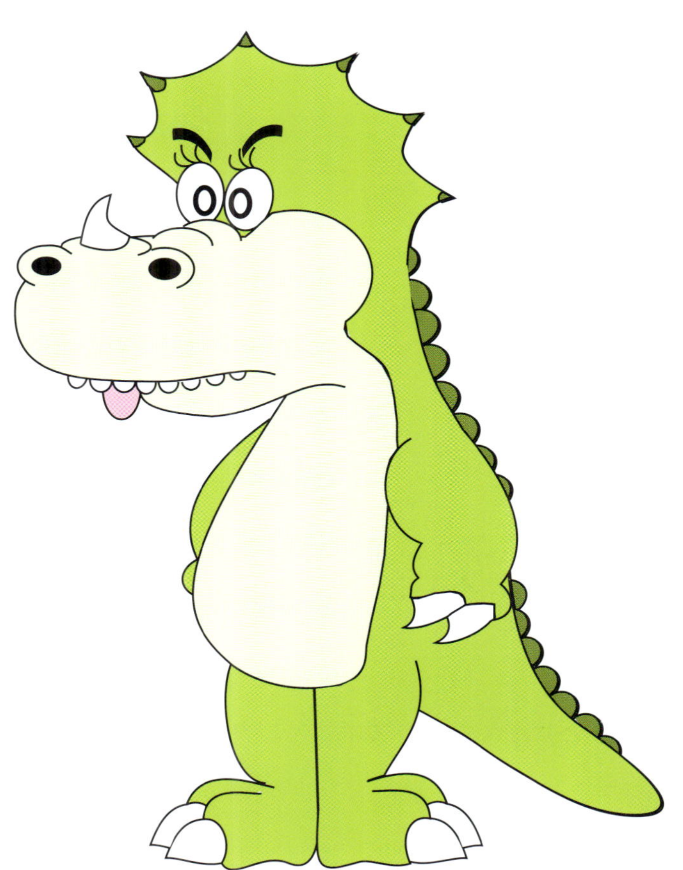

"*Morning* sickness?!" she scoffed,
"They did not get that right!"
She was queasy by sunrise but green by the night.

She tried gingersnaps, lemons,
And salty snack chips,
But all was repulsive that passed through her lips.

Her mood swings swung
Like an ape in the trees,
One minute fine, and then nothing could please.

Her sweet, patient man
Was incredibly kind,
But he secretly thought she was out of her mind!

He could never admit it
For fear of his life
But believed body-snatchers took over his wife.

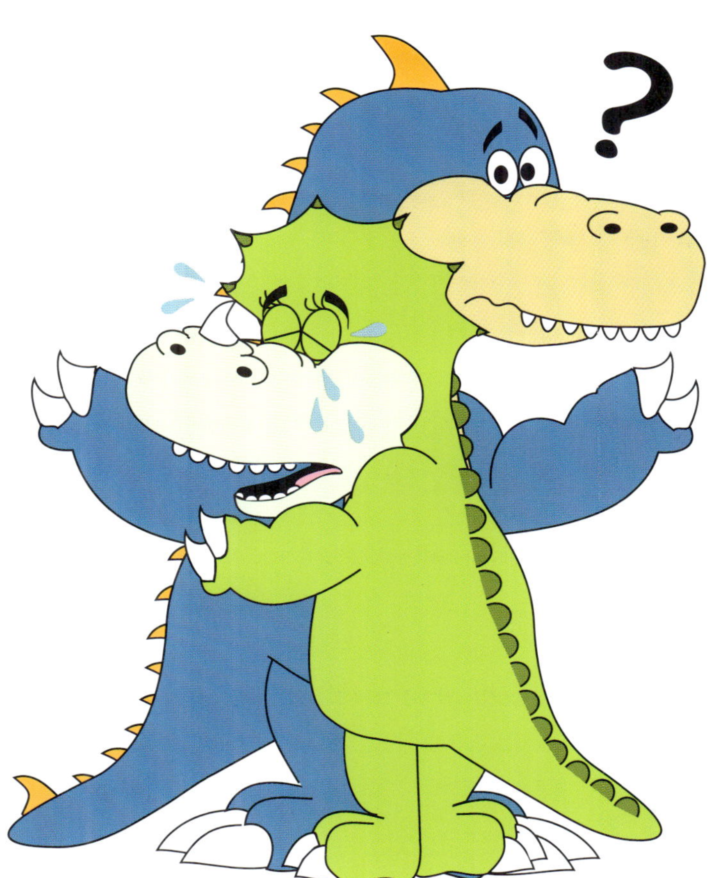

One late afternoon
She lay down for a nap,
And as she was drifting she felt a small tap.

The teeniest movement,
Just barely a flutter,
But she realized the source of this strange stomach stutter.

And she smiled
As the baby was suddenly real,
No longer a figment but flesh she could feel.

The fourth month went,
And left in its wake
A hunger so fierce it would just overtake.

With alarm
She noticed the growth of her gut
Was rivaled in size by her burgeoning butt!

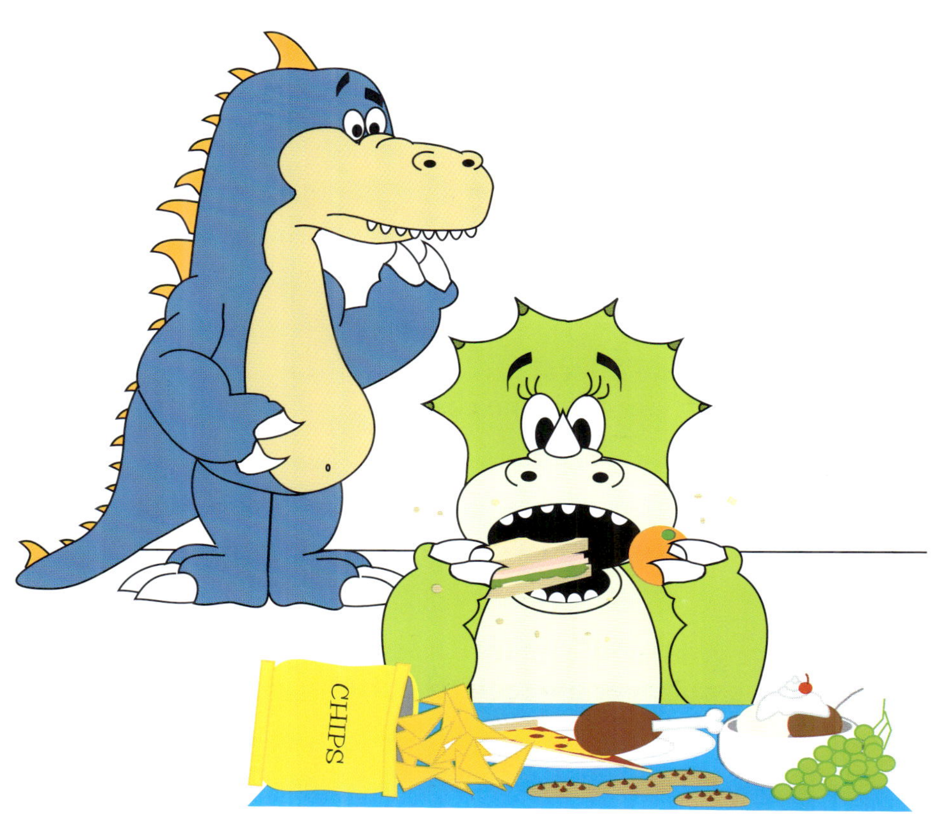
CHIPS

But every few hours
Her tum would implore
And it growled with a famine she couldn't ignore.

So she'd chomp and munch
And graze and crunch
An unceasing cycle of dinnerbreakfastlunch,

This caused heartburn
She readily came to despise,
It ignited her stomach, then started to rise.

She would visibly wince
As the acid blazed higher:
Esophagus raging from this inner fire.

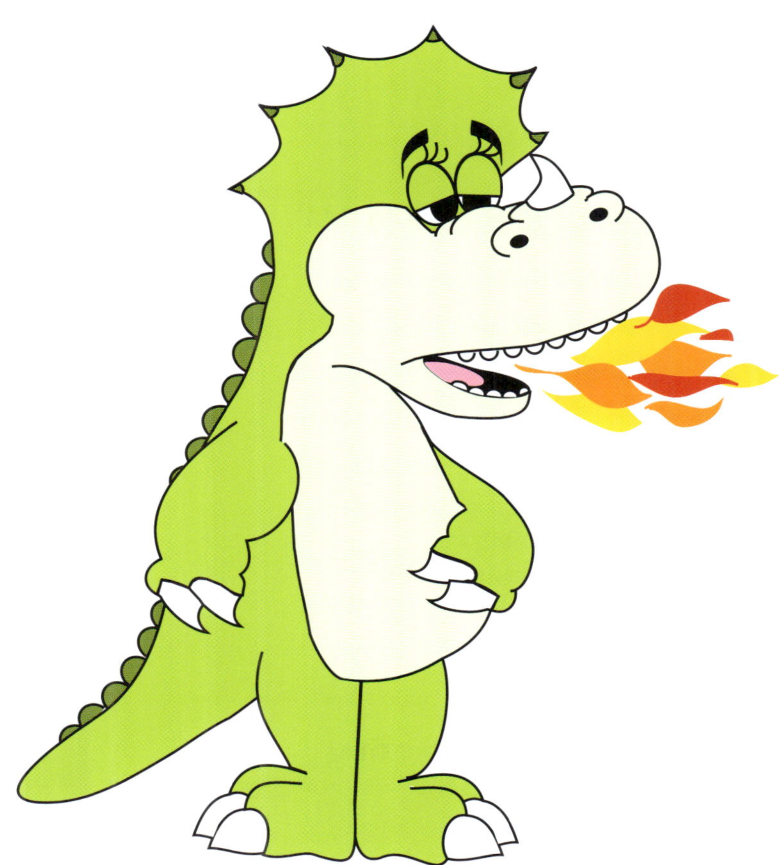

Her hair became
Healthier, fuller and long,
She was blissfully grateful that it grew so strong.

But she sensed that this gift
Would have come at a price,
And with pregnancy, nothing discreet would suffice.

It was peach-fuzz
That rooted all over the place,
On her stomach and arms and especially her face.

Her doctor assured her
It would go away,
But she felt like a downy sasquatch anyway.

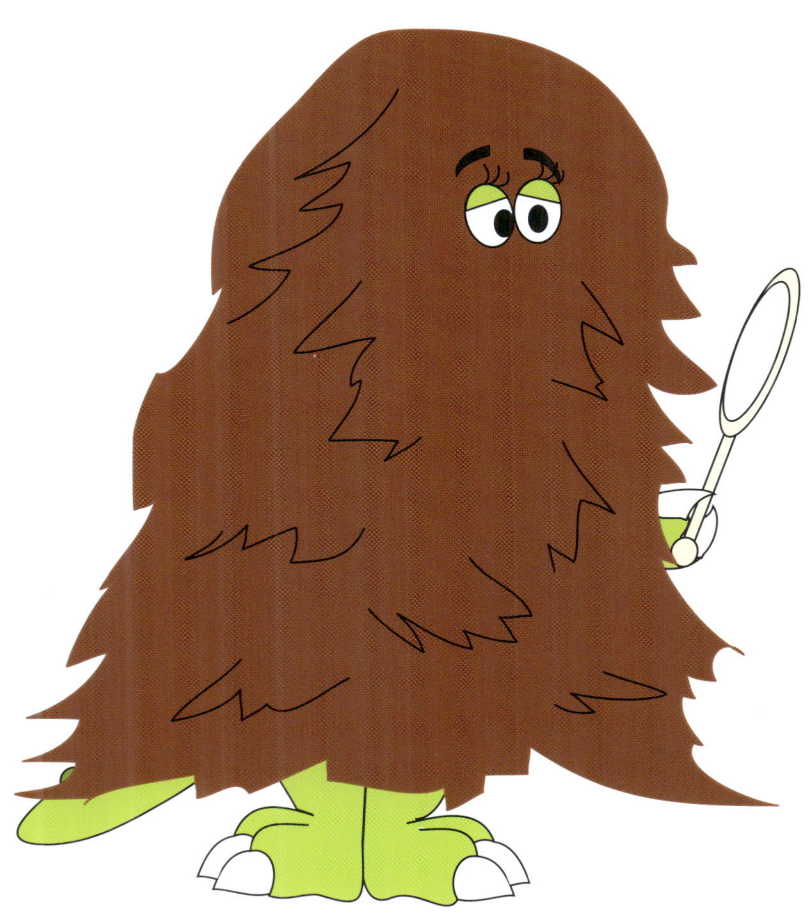

The most recent nuisance
Would wake her from slumber:
Her hip joints would seize up too often to number.

She'd stand up to
Stretch out this pelvic revolt
But her legs would give way like a newly born colt.

By each evening her ankles
Were puffy and round,
Reminiscent of pale tennis balls, she had found.

As her sock rings
Grew deeper with each passing day,
It was obvious the cankles were planning to stay.

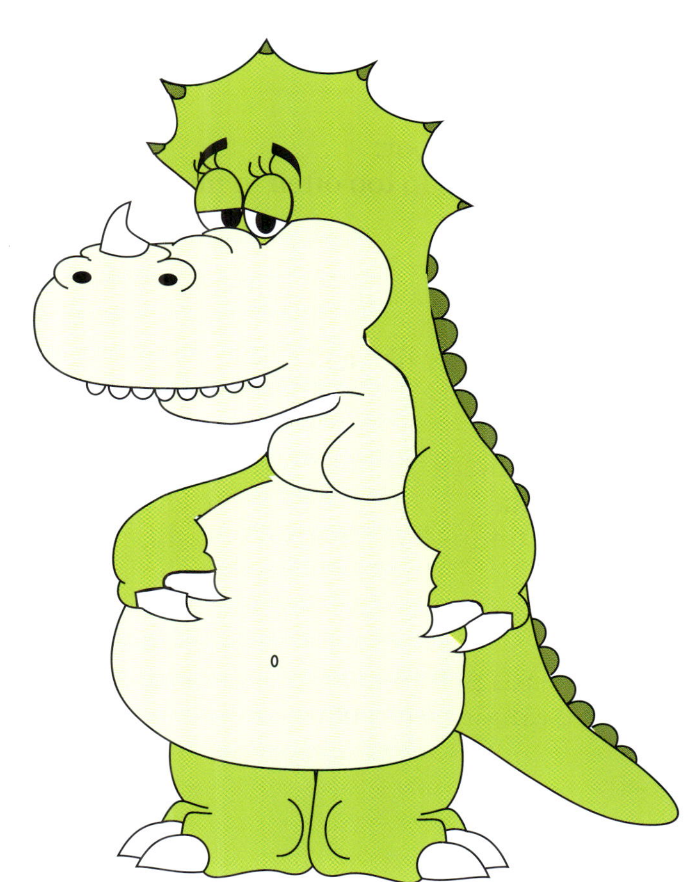

It was time to go shop
And acquire the "stuff,"
They had put off the purchase thereof long enough.

As they speechlessly wandered
The gadget-packed aisles,
There were walls of contraptions for mind-boggling miles.

Would they take the big stroller
For lapping the park?
Or succumb to the binky that glowed in the dark?

Did their eyes just deceive them?
Or could it be true?
An electric wipe warmer to mop baby's poo?!

It was simply astounding,
For someone so small:
They'd require a warehouse to capture it all!

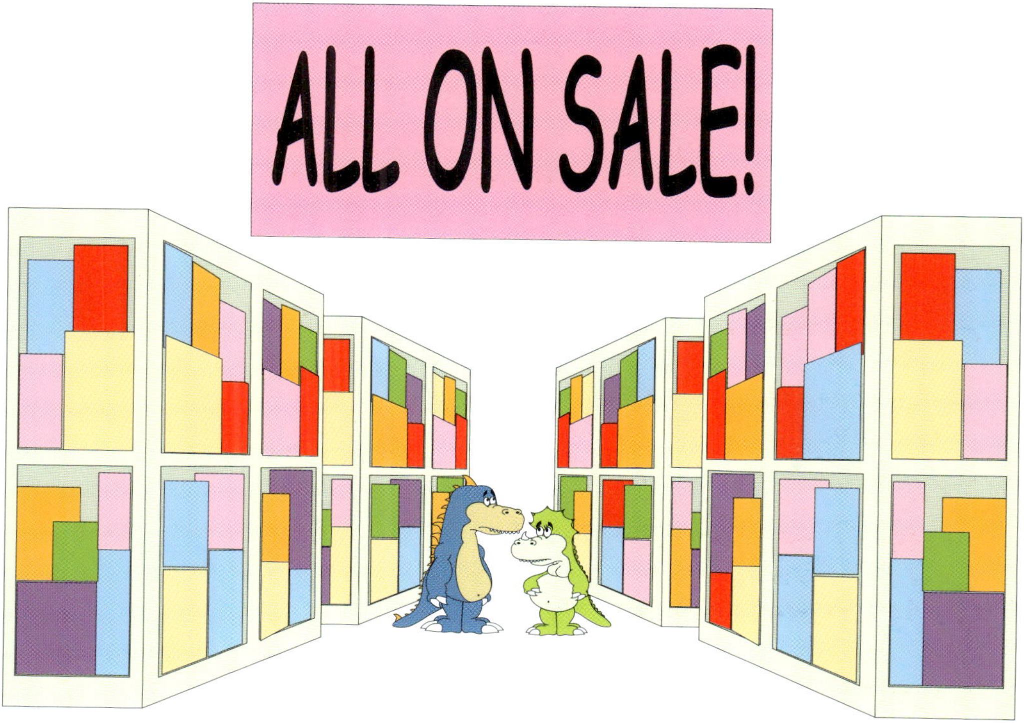

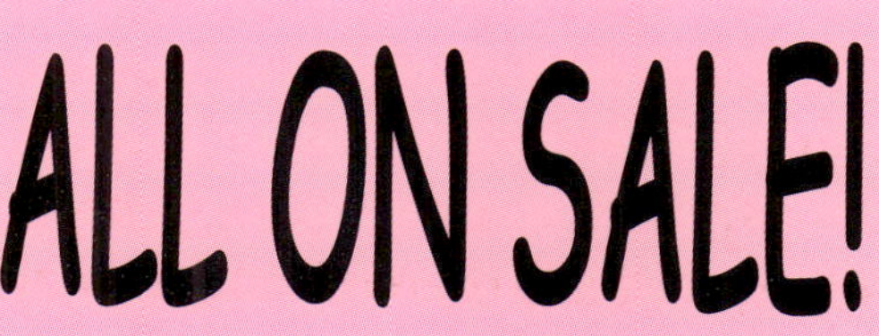
ALL ON SALE!

The Pregnasaurus was graceful no more,
Everything in her hands found its way to the floor,
And picking it up was a terrible chore.

Even something as simple
As turning in bed,
Became a five minute production instead.

She flopped and lolled
And heaved and rolled
And then wriggled some more for the pillows to mould.

There were five of them
Stationed at various points
To attempt to relieve her gelatinous joints.

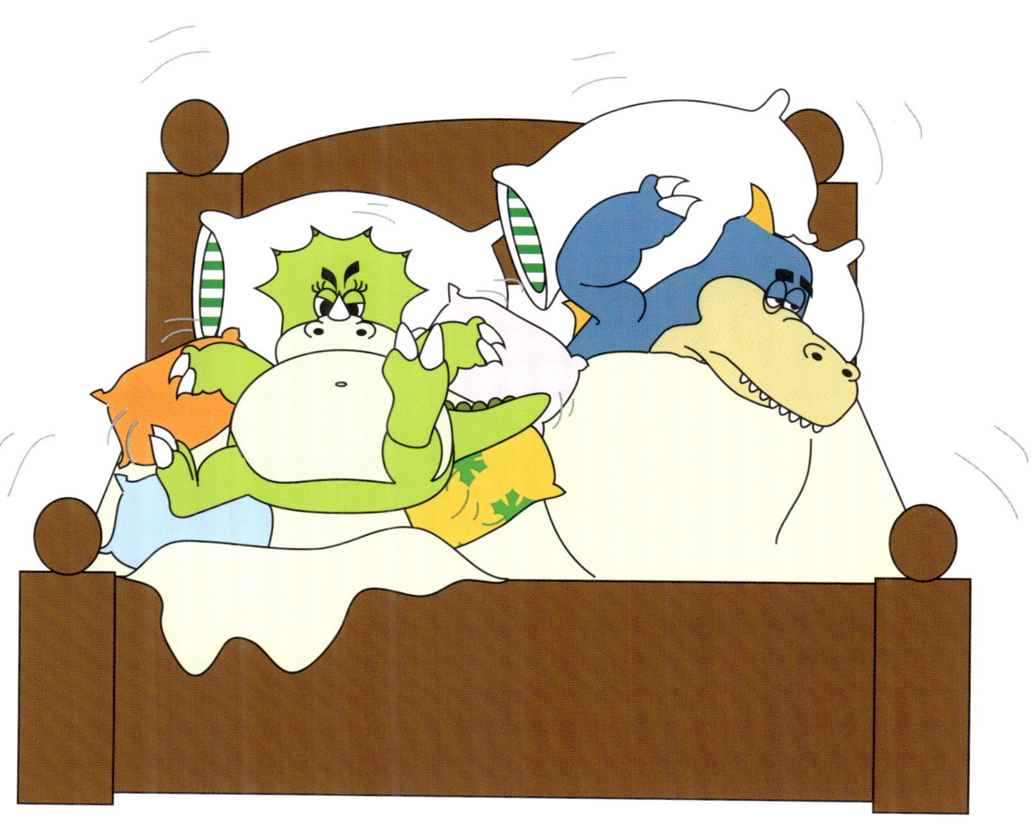

By the eighth month
Her belly protruded so far
That she barely fit in the front seat of her car.

Each day it got harder
To tie her shoelaces,
She grimaced and grunted and made funny faces.

Her sciatic nerve
Was the next to give out,
And it twinged in her back as she lumbered about.

Then horror of horrors,
She started to do
What she'd earnestly SWORN she would not give in to:

Her gait was transformed
From a graceful sway
To a waddlous display of a penguin sashay!

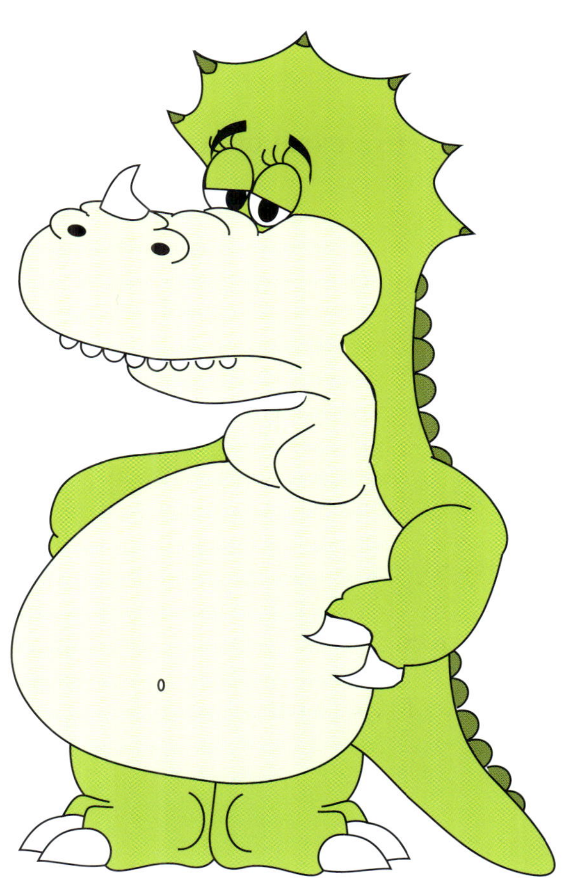

Her water-logged wrists
Caused her hands to go numb,
From her sausagey pinkie to tingley thumb.

Until thirty six weeks
Her taut skin was intact
But as forty approached it revealed a sad fact.

There were stretchmarks
Which burst like a juicy bratwurst
Leaving tiger striations she bitterly cursed.

An edema
Discovered at week thirty eight,
Had her sentenced to bed for the rest of the wait.

As she languished with boredom
She silently prayed
That the end of this journey would not be delayed.

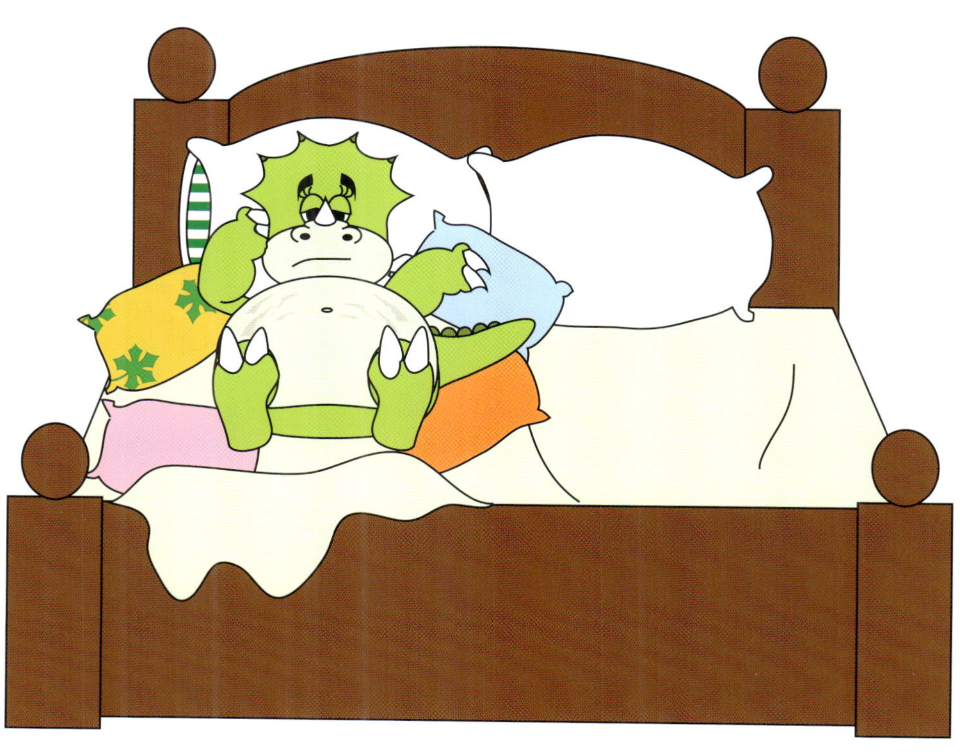

The contractions began
With a raging kick-start,
They appeared out of nowhere, two minutes apart.

They set off for the hospital
Keenly aware,
'Twas their last ride together as only a pair.

Modesty...Privacy...Dignity...
What?
These were relics her memory promptly forgot.

There were needles, IV bags,
And prodding and poking,
And monitoring heart rates and frequent pulse taking.

The doctor
Was not too convinced this was it,
He believed that her labor was not quite legit.

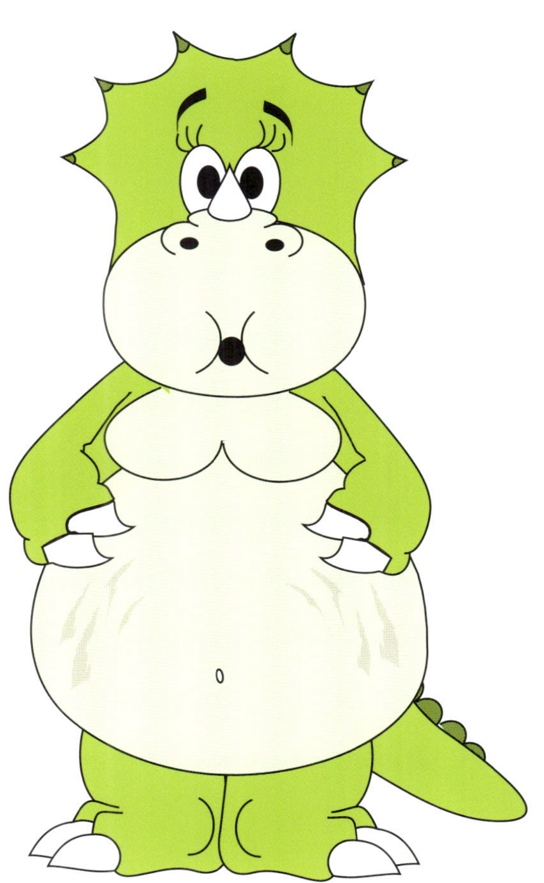

But as morning
Gave wearily way into noon,
The contractions kept coming and still just as soon.

So they called her best friend
Who got on the next flight,
And flew eight hundred miles to be with them that night.

Her friend and her husband
Took alternate shifts,
Helped her into the bathroom and brought her ice chips.

Over thirty four hours
Came and went,
The gut-wrenching contractions did not make a dent.

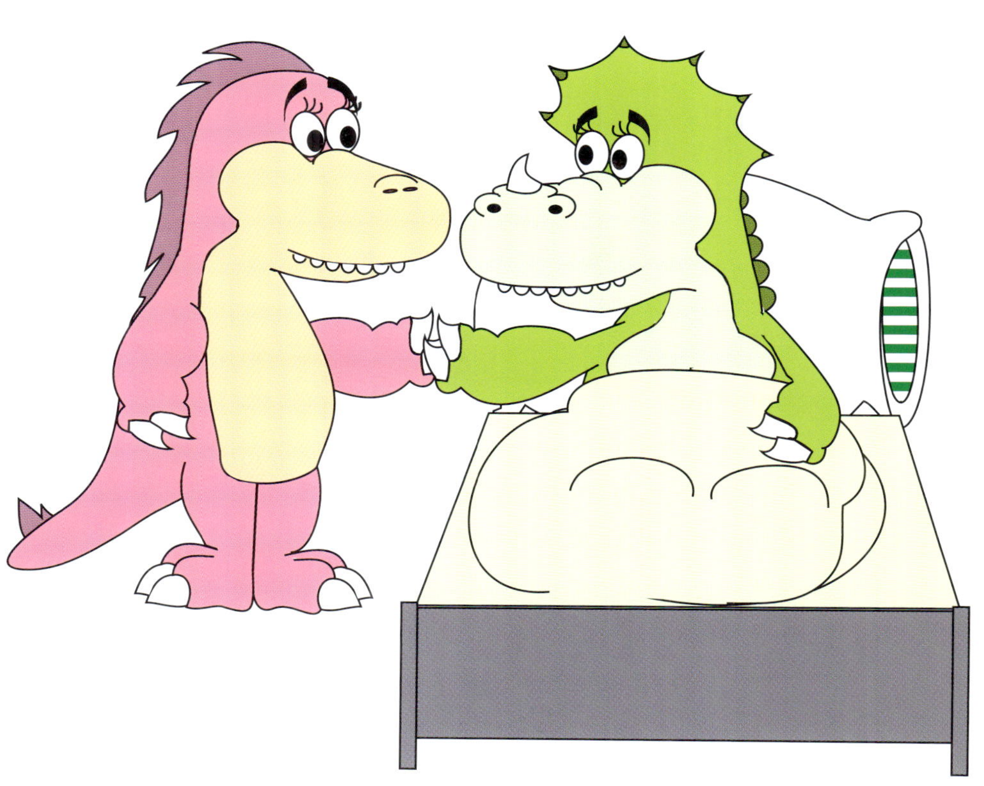

When they checked they assessed
That she hadn't progressed,
She had only reached two centimeters at best.

As the sixth bag of saline
Flowed into her vein
They determined the baby was feeling the strain.

They administered oxygen
Hoping to improve
The distressed baby's vitals but the stats didn't move.

She was starting to swell,
Her blood pressure to climb
Too late for induction, she'd run out of time.

They gave her a spinal
And prepped her C-Section
And performed other things too undignified to mention.

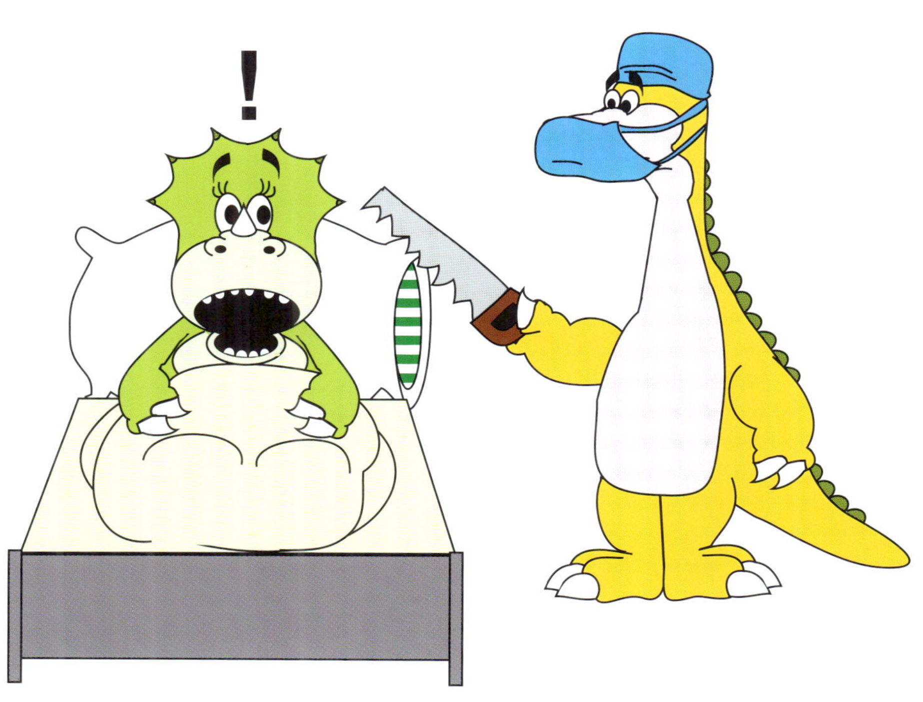

Only minutes elapsed
'Til they both heard the chorus,
The first cries of their brand new Babysaurus.

She had ten perfect fingers
And ten perfect toes,
And the silkiest skin and the buttonest nose.

She had whispery lashes
And tiny, sweet lips,
And the teeniest nails on her wee fingertips.

She had sapphire eyes
That were bright and alert,
And a set of plump cheeks they could eat for dessert.

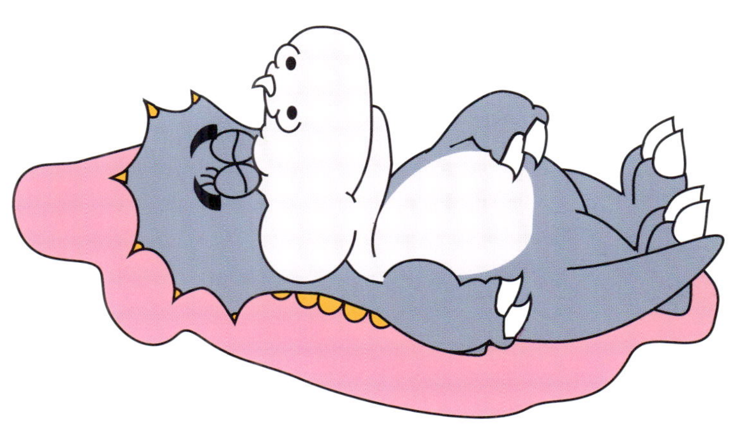

They had heard the cliché
That there aren't words to start,
To begin to describe what fills up in your heart.

But the truth is
No language on Earth can provide
Means to justly express the emotional tide.

They fell instantly,
Totally, madly in love
With their beautiful miracle sent from above.

For this perfect, small angel
She'd honestly vouch:
It was worth every moment, each ache and each ouch.

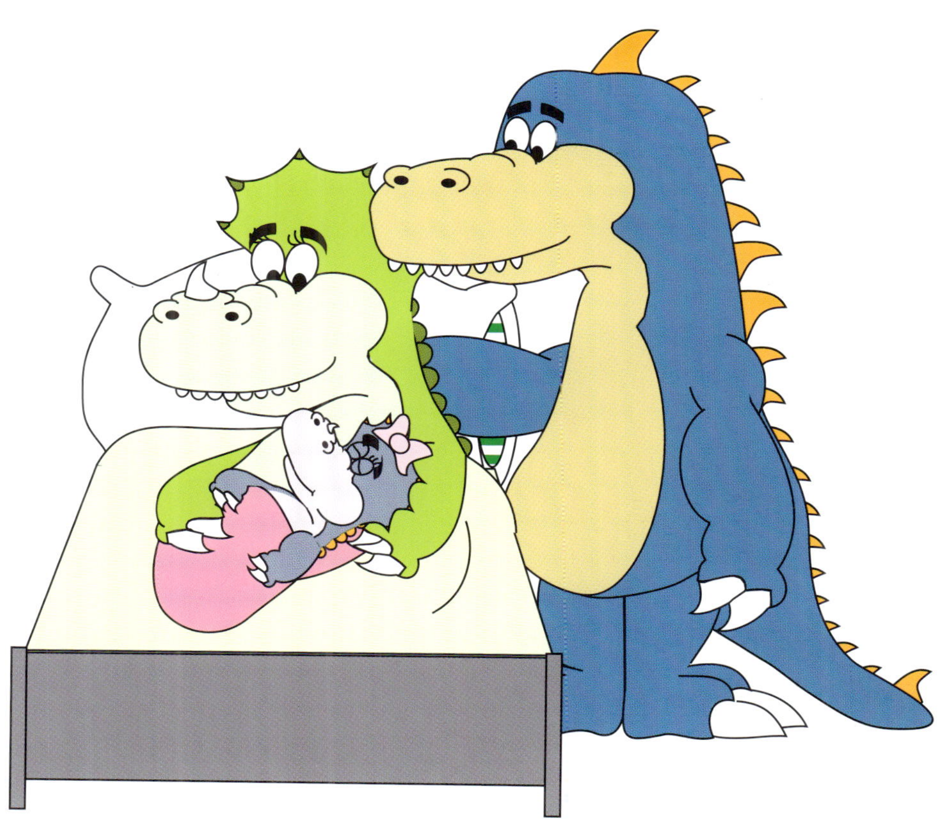